Home Health Aide Exam Prep

Home Care Aide Test Review

2nd Edition

Jane John-Nwankwo   RN, MSN

HOME HEALTH AIDE EXAM PREP: HOME CARE AIDE TEST REVIEW

2nd Edition

Copyright © 2015 by Jane John-Nwankwo RN, MSN

ISBN-13: 978-1514129395

ISBN-10: 1514129396

Printed in the United States of America.

OTHER TITLES FROM THE SAME AUTHOR:

1. Director of Staff Development: The Nurse Educator (2nd Edition)
2. CNA Exam Prep: Nurse Assistant Practice Test Questions. Vol. One (2nd Edition)
3. CNA Exam Prep: Nurse Assistant Practice Test Questions. Vol. Two (2nd Edition)
4. IV Therapy & Blood Withdrawal Review Questions
5. Medical Assistant Certification Study Guide Volume one & two
6. EKG Test Prep
7. Phlebotomy Test Prep
8. The Home Health Aide Textbook (2nd Edition)
9. How to make a million in nursing 2015
10. Personality Types
11. How to Become a Better Wife
12. How to Become a Better Husband
13. How to Grow Your Small Business
14. It's in Your Hands: 5 Strategies to Achieving Your Life Dreams (Best Seller)
15. Weight Loss Inspiration
16. How to Start Your Own business

Simply search "Jane John-Nwankwo" on Amazon!

www.djngbooks.org

www.janejohn-nwankwo.com

OTHER TITLES FROM THE SAME AUTHOR:

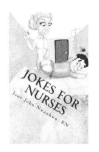 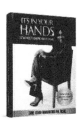 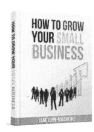 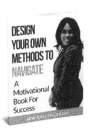 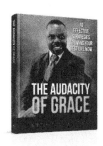

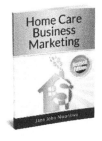 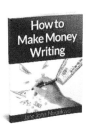 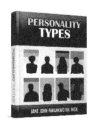 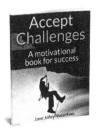

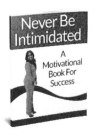 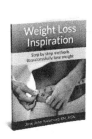 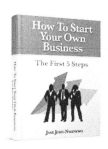 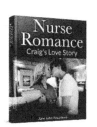

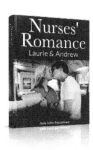 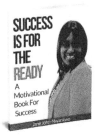 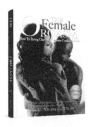 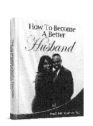 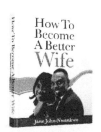

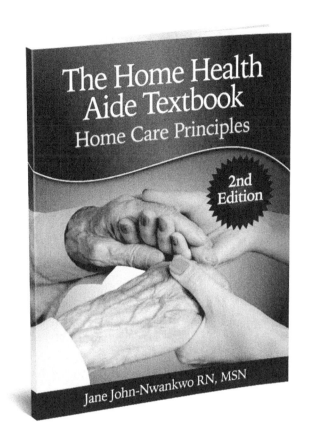

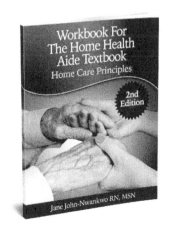

TABLE OF CONTENTS

1) ……………...provides assistance to the chronically ill, the elderly, and family caregivers who need relief from the stress of care-giving?

    A) Home health Aides

    B) Pastors

    C) Engineers

    D) Surgeons

2) Agencies pay home health aides from payments they receive from the following payers:

    A) Insurance companies

    B) Health maintenance organizations

    C) Medicare

    D) All of the above

3) The Centre for Medicare and Medicaid services payment system for home care is called the:

    A) Home health prospective payment system

    B) Pay per charge

    C) Service payment

    D) Medical payment

4) Clients who need home care are referred by a doctor to a:

    A) Hospital

    B) Friend

    C) Neighbor

    D) Home health agency

5) All home health aides are under supervision of one of the following skilled professionals:

    A) An engineer

    B) A pastor

C) A registered nurse

D) Native medicine

6) All of the following constitute the team of health professionals except:

A) Home health aides

B) Nurses

C) Doctors

D) Engineers

7) ………………helps clients learn to compensate for disabilities:

A) A client

B) An occupational therapist

C) Speech language pathologist

D) Registered dietitian

8) A legal term that means someone can be held responsible for harming someone else is referred to as:

A) Assets

B) Liability

C) Action

D) Discipline

9) A particular method, or way, of doing something is called:

A) Orientation

B) A procedure

C) An activity

D) Information

10) A professional relationship with a client includes:

A) Maintaining a negative attitude

B) Not finishing assignments

C) Doing only the tasks assigned

D) None of the above

11) Professionalism means:

A) Having to do with work or a job

B) Your life outside your job

C) Disapproving client's opinion

D) Keeping late to work

12) ……………teaches clients and their families about special diets to improve their health and help them manage their illness:

A) A medical social worker

B) A registered dietitian

C) An occupational therapist

D) None of the above

13) A professional relationship with an employer does not include of the following:

A) Always being on time

B) Completing assignments efficiently

C) Maintaining a negative attitude

D) Participating in education programs offered

14) Which of the following depicts the meaning of laws?

A) Laws are rules set by the government

B) Laws tell us what we must do

C) Laws help to ensure order and safety

D) All of the above

15) ……………defines the things you are allowed to do and describes how to do them correctly:

A) A plan

B) A liability

C) A procedure

D) A scope of practice

16) Which of the following is not an example of legal and ethical behavior by HHAs?

A) Protecting client's privacy

B) Accepting gifts and tips

C) Being honest at all times

D) Documenting accurately and promptly

17) Clients have the right to:

A) Have access, upon request, to all bills for service the client has received

B) Receive care of the highest quality

C) Refuse services without fear of reprisal

D) All of the above

18) Unexplained injuries including burns, bruises, and bone injuries can be referred to as:

A) Mental abuse

B) Physical abuse

C) Psychological abuse

D) Passive neglect

19) You can help protect your client's rights in which of the following ways:

A) Respect your clients' property

B) Talk or gossip about a client

C) Neglect clients in your planning

D) Enter a client's room without knocking and seeking permission

20) To respect confidentiality means:

A) To tell the a client's best friend about his friend's health condition

B) To keep private things secret

C) To discuss issues about a client with in a family meeting

D) None of the above

21) ………………..is the process of exchanging information with others:

A) Looking

B) Recreation

C) Communication

D) Interpretation

22) Always report combative behaviors of clients to your:

A) Parents

B) Client's friend

C) Friend

D) Supervisor

23) All of the following are some barriers to communication, except:

A) Client hears and understands you clearly

B) Client is difficult to understand

C) Asking why

D) Client speaking in a different language

24) Which of the following questions would you ask a client for adequate clarifications?

A) Did you sleep last night?

B) Did he rape you?

C) Tell me about your sleep last night

D) Is exercise good?

25) Reasons for documentation include:

A) It guarantees clear and complete communication

B) It provides up-to-date record of the status of a client

C) Documentation protects you and the employer from liability

D) All of the above

26) File an incident report when one of the following incidents occurs:

    A) You client performs an exercise

    B) Your client falls

    C) When a patient is safe

    D) When a client lies on the right side of the body

27) The process of removing pathogens or state of being free from pathogens is referred to as:

    A) Medical asepsis

    B) Plasmodiasis

    C) Sepsis

    D) Toxoplasmosis

28) …………..is where the pathogen lives and grows:

    A) House

    B) Ecosystem

    C) Landscape

    D) Reservoir

29) An uninfected person who could get sick or infected is referred to as a:

    A) Portal of entry

    B) Causative agent

    C) Susceptible host

    D) Sepsis

30) If blood or body fluid spills on fabrics such as carpets and clothes:

    A) Use alcohol to clean it

    B) Use commercial disinfectants to clean it

    C) Clean with bleach

    D) None of the above

31) ………………..is a federal government agency that issues information to protect the health of individuals and communities:

A) Health firm

B) World health organization

C) The centre for disease control and prevention

D) Individual co-operations

32) One of the following is not included as one of the measures of standard precautions:

A) Clean a client's blood without wearing gloves

B) Wash your hands before putting on gloves

C) Wear gloves if you may come in contact with body fluids

D) Wear a disposable gown that is resistant to body fluid

33)………………...refers to washing hands with water and soap or other detergents that contain an antiseptic agent:

A) Hand antisepsis

B) Hand rinsing

C) Protocols

D) None of the above

34) Equipment that helps protect employees from serious injuries or illnesses resulting from contact with workplace hazards is called:

A) Personal protective equipment

B) Standard precaution

C) Hospital policy

D) Health machineries

35) Personal protective equipment includes the following, except one:

A) Masks

B) Goggles

C) Gowns

D) Needles

36) One of the following is not an airborne disease:

A) Measles

B) Tuberculosis

C) Boil

D) Chickenpox

37) Droplets can be created by:

A) Coughing

B) Sneezing

C) Laughing

D) All of the above

38) An example of a droplet disease is the:

A) Rash

B) Scabies

C) Mumps

D) Constipation

39) MRSA stands for:

A) Menstrual reluctant stage of Action

B) Men Rehabilitation system activities

C) Methicillin-resistant staphylococcus aureas

D) None of the above

40) Droplet precautions include:

A) Wearing a face mask during care

B) Restricting visits from uninfected people

C) An infected client covering his nose and mouth with a tissue when sneezing

D) All of the above

41) The way the parts of the body works together whenever you move is referred to as:

A) Body mechanics

B) Movement

C) Body structure

D) Matrix

42) When you stand, your weight is centered in:

A) Elbows

B) Your arms

C) Your pelvis

D) Fibula

43) Disorientation means confusion about:

A) Person

B) Place

C) Time

D) All of the above

44) Burns can be caused by one of the following:

A) Cold water

B) Hand shaking

C) Dry heat

D) Waxing floors

45) Employee's responsibilities for infection control include the following:

A) Follow standard precautions

B) Take advantage of the free hepatitis B vaccination

C) Immediately report any exposure you have to infection, or blood

D) All of the above

46) One of the following is not a guideline to guide against fire:

   A) Stay in or near the kitchen when anything is cooking

   B) Discourage careless smoking and smoking in bed

   C) Turn on heaters when no one is home

   D) Do not leave dryer on when you leave the house

47) To ensure travel safety:

   A) Avoid planning your route

   B) Use turn signals

   C) Encourage distractions from friends

   D) Drive without seat belt

48) Factors that raise the risk for falls include:

   A) Clutter

   B) Slippery floors

   C) Poor lighting

   D) All of the above

49) …………..is emergency care given immediately to an injured person?

   A) Exercise

   B) Head stretching

   C) 9111

   D) First aid

50) The first signs of insulin reaction include one of the following:

   A) Pneumonia

   B) Heart failure

   C) Constipation

   D) Nervousness

51) All human beings have the same basic physical needs which include:

A) Food and water

B) Activity

C) Sleep and rest

D) All of the above

52) One of the following is not a psychosocial need:

A) Love and affection

B) Shelter

C) Security

D) Self esteem

53) A system of learned behaviors, practiced by a group of people that are considered to be the tradition of that people is called:

A) Actualization

B) Tribe

C) Culture

D) Precision

54) ………..is the name for the condition in which all of the body's systems are their best?

A) Homeostasis

B) Metabolism

C) Peristalsis

D) Arthritis

55) Which of the following is not a system of the body?

A) Endocrine system

B) Diving system

C) Urinary system

D) Nervous system

56) When the outside temperature is too high, the blood vessels:

A) Constrict

B) Becomes excited

C) Dilate

D) Shortens

57) Which of the following gives the body shape and structure?

A) Apocrine and eccrine structures

B) Veins

C) Arteries

D) Bones and ligaments

58) The nervous system controls and coordinates all body functions.

A) True

B) False

59) The taking-in (breathing in) of oxygen by the body is referred to as:

A) Inspiration

B) Expiration

C) Purification

D) Exchange

60) The largest system organ and the system in the body are the:

A) Mouth

B) Skin

C) Esophagus

D) The small intestine

61) One of the following is a common musculoskeletal system disorder?

A) Nephrotic syndrome

B) Histoplasmosis

C) Pneumonia

D) Osteoporosis

62) The digestive system is also called:

A) Respiratory system

B) Digestive system

C) Metabolic system

D) Nervous system

63) The two major functions of gastrointestinal system are:

A) Digestion and elimination

B) Digestion and locomotion

C) Elimination and respiration

D) None of the above

64) Endocrine glands secrete:

A) Hormones

B) Enzymes

C) Lipase

D) Amylase

65) The sex cells are formed in the male and female sex glands called the:

A) Gonads

B) Androgens

C) Estrogens

D) Lymphatic

66) At age 1-3 toddlers learn to:

A) Choose education

B) Speak

C) Prepare for retirement

D) Develop language skills and vocabularies

67) ……………is a disease or condition that will eventually cause death?

A) A recuperating disease

B) An acute condition

C) Reproductive system

D) A terminal disease

68) The term for the special care a dying person needs is called?

A) Skin care

B) Hospice care

C) Recuperation

D) Advancement stage

69) Which of the following is not included in the normal changes of aging?

A) Incontinence

B) Immunity weakens

C) Appetite decreases

D) Short-term memory loss occurs

70) Common disorders found in infancy period include:

A) Prematurity

B) Low birth weight

C) Sudden infant death syndrome

D) All of the above

71) Which of the following are the basic body positions?

A) Supine

B) Lateral

C) Prone

D) All of the above

72) One of the most important things to consider when transferring a client to a chair or a bed is:

A) Safety

B) Nutrition

C) The Family

D) Finance

73) Contractures are generally caused by:

A) Exercise

B) Driving

C) Locomotion

D) Immobility

74) Pulling a client across sheets can cause:

A) Fluid retention

B) Shearing

C) Spinal cord damage

D) None of the above

75) …………….is a device, such as splint or a brace, which helps support and align a limb and improve its functioning?

A) Leaning table

B) An orthotic device

C) Hand role

D) Head pillows

76) Hygiene and grooming activities, as well as dressing, eating and toileting are called?

A) Activities of daily living

B) Recreational activities

C) Indoor activities

D) Unhealthy life styles

77) Oral care should be performed at least:

A) Once a day

B) At bed time

C) Twice a day

D) None of the above

78) ……………is the inhalation of food, fluid or foreign material into the lungs?

A) Expiration

B) Inspiration

C) Aspiration

D) Asphyxia

79) Moving a body part towards the midline of the body is referred to as:

A) Supination

B) Phonation

C) Rotation

D) Adduction

80) One of the following is not done if a client starts to fall during a transfer?

A) Try to reverse or stop a fall

B) Widen your stance

C) Call for help if a family member is around

D) Do not try to reverse or stop a fall

81)……………is the impairment of physical or mental functions:

A) A disability

B) Burn

C) Neuralgia

D) Heart failure

82) A fallacy is:

A) An opinion

B) Truth

C) Being sure

D) A false belief

83) Which of the following can cause mental illness or make it worse?

A) Heredity

B) Stress

C) Environmental factors

D) All of the above

84) Sadness is the only one symptom of:

A) Happiness

B) Depression

C) Hopefulness

D) Excitement

85) Arthritis causes:

A) Dementia

B) Tuberculosis

C) Constipation

D) Stiffness and pain

86) In diabetes mellitus, the pancreas does not produce enough:

A) Estrogen

B) Prolactin

C) Insulin

D) Progesterone

87) Type 2 diabetes can also be referred to as:

A) Adult-onset diabetes

B) Electrically-charged insufficiency

C) Childbearing diabetes

D) All of the above

88) Paralysis on one side of the body is called:

A) Hemiplegia

B) Aphasia

C) Quadriplegia

D) Dysphagia

89) Risk factors for cancer include the following, except:

A) Poor nutrition

B) Water

C) Radiation

D) Tobacco use

90) A brain disorder that affects a person's ability to think and communicate clearly is called:

A) Anemia

B) AIDS

C) Paresis

D) Schizophrenia

91) Which of the following practices are accepted during housekeeping?

A) Be organized when performing tasks

B) Main a safe environment

C) Familiarize yourself with the household's cleaning materials

D) All of the above

92) Cleaning of the kitchen should be done:

A) Once a day

B) At night only

C) After every use

D) Once in a week

93) Which of the following is an example of a detergent?

A) Soap

B) Iodine

C) Kerosene

D) Anion

94) The process of giving special treatment to items that have heavy soil, spots,, and stains before washing them is called:

A) Retreating

B) Escalation

C) Retouching

D) Pretreating

95) Which of the following would be the reason for changing bed linens?

A) The sheets are wrinkled, making a client uncomfortable

B) The linen was used by another client

C) The linen is damp or unclean

D) All of the above

96) The process by which nutrients are broken down to be used by the body for energy and other needs is referred to as:

A) Reproduction

B) Metabolism

C) Excitation

D) Lyses

97) There are …………..nutrients needed by the body for growth and development:

A) Three

B) Two

C) Six

D) Four

98) Foods high in sodium include the following, except:

A) Bacon

B) Ham

C) Sausage

D) Orange

99) The state of being frightened, excited, confused, in danger or irritated is referred to as:

A) Stress

B) Joy

C) Mood change

D) None of the above

100)…………..occurs when a person does not have enough fluid in his body?

A) Dehydration

B) Fluid overload

C) Crackles in the lungs

D) Water toxicity

Section Two

1. The ideal caregiver is someone who knows his/her responsibilities, maintain punctuality very open to suggestions and takes pride in his/her job

   A. True

   B. False

   C. Neither

2. The responsibilities of the caregiver include all of the following except

   A. Routine personal care hygiene assistance

   B. Prescribing medications

   C. Rides to doctor appointments and errands

3. _____ is define as skillfulness by virtue a possessing special knowledge

   A. Limitations

   B. Identification

   C. Professionalism

4. A caregiver should always wear tight fitting jeans or pants to work

   A. True

   B. False

   C. Neither

5. Should you maintain personal hygiene as a caregiver

   A. Sometimes

   B. Always

   C. Never

6. _____ means the quality or habit of adhering to an appointed time

   A. Responsibility

   B. Professional

   C. Punctuality

7. If you find your patient slump all of a sudden while eating at the dining table what should you do?

   A. Call 911, start CPR, call your agency

   B. Run

   C. Just ignore your patient because you are just there to make money

8. An ideal caregiver does not adjust to the needs of the patient

   A. True

   B. False

   C. Neither

9. Some problems that could occur when caregivers put themselves last include all of the following except

   A. Meeting their own needs

   B. They become ill and hate their job

   C. They do not deliver appropriate care to their patient

10. The United States made three 12 hour shifts full time to burn out caregivers

    A. True

    B. False

    C. Neither

11. If you want to be an ideal care giver then you need to stay in good health

    A. True

    B. False

    C. Neither

12. As a caregiver you should keep your own self updates about the disability or disease of the patient

   A. True

   B. False

   C. Neither

13. Bad communication is believed to be the most viable quality of a caregiver

   A. True

   B. False

   C. Neither

14. The 3 areas involve in keeping yourself safe as a caregiver involve all of the following except

   A. The five senses

   B. Information, sexual behaviors

   C. Interrogating the patient

15. Some of the signs of frustration are

   A. Feeling happy

   B. Singing all the time

   C. Headache, knot in throat, desire to strike out

16. Calming down is necessary when there are any tensed situations involving the patient

   A. True

   B. False

   C. Neither

17. Any uncontrollable situations should be dealt with right away

   A. True

   B. False

   C. Neither

18. Some common ways of decreasing your stress involves all of the following except

A. Meeting physical needs

B. Praise your self

C. Going on a romantic date with your patient

19. Bad communication with the patient or to someone related with the patient is not important

A. True

B. False

C. Neither

20. _____ communication is a form of expressing that is ineffective and maladaptive

A. Passive communication

B. Aggressive communication

C. Good communication

21. The most effective and healthiest form of communication is the _____ style

A. Aggressive

B. Passive

C. Assertive

22. Assertive style of communication is the style people use most

A. True

B. False

C. Neither

23. There are _____ communication technique which can help get your message across towards the

patient

A. 3

B. 5

C. 7

24. The first and foremost thing is to put our selves in their shoes

A. True

B. False

C. Neither

25. Listening carefully and respectfully to the values and beliefs of the patients and respecting them in your day to day activity is what is referred to as

    A. Cultural activity

    B. Assessment sensitivity

    C. Cultural sensitivity

26. _____ is referred to as the way of life of the people

    A. Norms

    B. Culture

    C. Beliefs

27. Advantages of cultural sensitivity involves all of the following except

    A. Avoidance of conflicts

    B. A stronger connection with the client and the family members

    C. Respecting your own feelings, desires and needs

28. Communication is not the best way to negotiate with any differences arising out of cultural sensitivity

    A. True

    B. False

    C. Neither

29. Escorting a patient should not be confused with accompanying a patient to a destination

    A. True

    B. False

    C. Neither

30. A person who is escorting and transporting a patient should not be aware of the medical history and the clinical condition of the patient

A. True

B. False

C. Neither

31. Some of the probable reasons of a fire breakout are smoking, cooking and a couple of other fire hazards

A. True

B. False

C. Neither

32. The battery of the alarms needs to be charged at least _____ in a year

A. Twice

B. Checked

C. Once

33. Politeness and simplicity is the only manners needed in conducting proper phone etiquette

A. True

B. False

C. Neither

34. With aging the risk for falling increases because their senses dim and nervous systems tends to deteriorate

A. True

B. False

C. Neither

35. It is true that most of the falls lead to minor injuries, but at the same time nearly _____ to _____ percent lead to fractures as well as other serious injuries

A. Ten, sixty

B. Ten, fifty

C. Ten, seventy

36. Injuries that can result out of falls are broken bones, head injuries and even accidents that harm the interior body parts

    A. True

    B. False

    C. Neither

37. _____ is a common form of dementia in which a person faces problem with their memory or thought process

    A. Lupus

    B. COPD

    C. Alzheimer's

38. The symptoms of Alzheimer's are divided in two categories: _____ stage and _____ stage

    A. Late, noon

    B. Early, late

    C. Early, evening

39. The emotional support needs to come from the side of the caregiver and this can create a sense of wellbeing in the patient

    A. True

    B. False

    C. Neither

40. The early stage of Alzheimer attacks the patient so badly that they are not even in a position to communicate properly and they are completely dependent on the caregiver

    A. True

    B. False

    C. Neither

41. Memory loss in the Alzheimer's disease doesn't mean that the patient loses their feelings

    A. True

B. False

C. Neither

42. The last stage of Alzheimer's completely cripples a person both mentally as well as physically

   A. True

   B. False

   C. Neither

43. _____ is a brain disorder that deals with an abnormal self-absorption with oneself

   A. Alzheimer's

   B. Mad cow

   C. Autism

44. Autistic children tend to play repetitive games with toys for example lining up of objects and the turning on and off of light switches despite repeated scolding

   A. True

   B. False

   C. Neither

45. Some physical characteristic of autism may include

   A. They are neat and well behave

   B. They communicate with adults only

   C. The skin is pale, face has low muscle tone

46. There is laboratory tests to confirm autism

   A. True

   B. False

   C. Neither

47. The autistic patient may have fixations like making repeated noises, staring at turning wheels etc.

   A. True

B. False

C. Neither

48. Autistic individuals often have good auditory processing skills

   A. True

   B. False

   C. Neither

49. The high functioning autistic adults are very successful and they live relatively normal lives

   A. True

   B. False

   C. Neither

50. The _____ adult autistics need constant care and attention like autistic children

   A. Low functioning

   B. High function

   C. Normal functioning

Section Three

1. How many hours in length are most Home Health Aide entry- level programs?

   a. 50

   b. 80

   c. 75

2. The person receiving care at home is called a ……….

    a. Patient

    b. Client

    c. Employee

3. The classroom portion of the Home Health Aide training usually consists of…….. hours (This differs from state to state)

    a. 60

    b. 50

    c. 40

4. Practicing the skills learned in the classroom in a client care setting is called……

    a. Evaluation

    b. Clinical experience

    c. Internship

5. How many hours are usually spent in a clinical experience for the Home Care Aide training?

    a. 20

    b. 25

    c. 15

6. This is the usual function of a person………….

    a. Role

    b. Ethnic

    c. Position

7. In the PQRST method, what does the P stand for?

    a. Patient

    b. Preview

    c. Prepare

8. Recognition by a government or nongovernment agency that a person has met certain requirements is ……………..

    a. Entry level

    b. Accomplishment

    c. Certification

9. A client's private information not to be discussed is called…………….

    a. HIPPA

    b. Secrets

    c. Protected health information

10. Process of judging employee performance to determine suitability to remain in the job is called

    a. Evaluation

    b. Role

    c. Ethnic

11. This is a federal program of hospitalization and health care insurance for persons older than 65 and/ or those with permanent disabilities

    a. Medicaid

    b. Medicare

    c. HMO insurance

12. This is a list of specific diagnoses used to determine the typical length of stay and the cost of treatment allowed for patients with that particular group of illness

    a. Hospice

    b. Standard

    c. Diagnosis- related group(DRG)

13. This is the state and federal insurance program that pays for hospitalization and health care for low- income persons of all ages

    a. Medicaid

    b. Medicare

    c. PPO insurance

14. Gauge that is used as a basis for judgment

    a. Policy

    b. Standard

    c. Behavior

15. Illness with a rapid onset and severe symptoms and of short length is called..............

    a. Illness

    b. Chronic illness

    c. Acute illness

16. Disease with a little change and slow progress and long of duration

    a. Acute illness

    b. Hospice

    c. Chronic illness

17. A program of care that assists the dying client to maintain a satisfactory lifestyle during the end

    stage of an illness

    a. Hospice

    b. Acute illness

    c. Chronic illness

18. A person who arranges for the care of a patient on release from the hospital is...........

    a. Doctor

    b. Hospital discharge planner

    c. Planner

19. In what year did the U.S. congress pass the Medicare law?

    a. 1995

    b. 1965

c. 1975

20. When a person has reached the highest level of ability after injury or accident but still needs assistance with routine care and therapy at home, this care is called..........

    a. Hospice

    b. Hospitals

    c. Rehabilitation

21. The sharing of thoughts, information, and opinions with others is called ....

    a. Communication

    b. Ethics

    c. Verbal communication

22. How many parts are involved in the process of communications?

    a. 2

    b. 3

    c. 4

23. Communications using the spoken word is known as...........

    a. Communications

    b. Verbal communications

    c. Telecommunications

24. This is the exchange of information without using words.............

    a. Telecommunications

    b. Nonverbal communications

    c. Communications

25. To like or dislike someone or something without a good reason is called...........

    a. Bias

    b. Grievance

    c. Ethics

26. Physical, mental, or emotional condition that interferes with abilities to carry out activities of daily living

    a. Surrogate

    b. Grievance

    c. Disability

27. The code of behavior or conduct is called………..

    a. Verbal communication

    b. Ethics

    c. Confidentiality

28. Good listening involves the use of eyes, ears, and feelings

    a. T

    b. F

29. What are the four parts in the process of communication?

    a. Sender, receiver, message, and feedback

    b. Receiver, message, sender, listener

    c. Listener, sender, message, feedback

30. In home care, communication is the link between you, the client, and the agency

    a. T

    b. F

31. This is defined as a requirement for survival……….

    a. Self- esteem

    b. Need

    c. Want

32. Pertaining to the normal functioning of the body is ………….

    a. Peers

    b. Need

c. Physiological

33. Who provides most of the care early in one's life?

   a. Primary caregiver

   b. Nurse

   c. Doctor

34. Thinking and feeling good about yourself is called…………

   a. Self- actualization

   b. Need

   c. Self- esteem

35. Who described the basic human needs and used a pyramid shape to illustrate them?

   a. Diagnosis- related group

   b. Abraham Maslow

   c. HIPPA

36. What is listed at the base of the pyramid (highest priority?

   a. Self- actualization

   b. Love

   c. Physiological

37. This is the state of reaching one's full potential and being able to cope with problems.

   a. Self- actualization

   b. Self- esteem

   c. Security and safety

38. What does it mean when one belongs to a nuclear family?

   a. Uncles, nephews and aunties

   b. Father, mother and children

   c. A circle of friends

39. When one belongs to a family of procreation, it means……………

a. A group of people who live together

b. The family we have started

c. Single and living alone

40. How many major stages are there in human growth and development?

a. 7

b. 10

c. 15

41. …………… is the construction and arrangements of cells, tissues, organs, and organ system

a. Systematic organ

b. Atrophy

c. Body structure

42. This is the basic functioning unit of the body and are the smallest structures of all living things.

a. Tissues

b. Cells

c. Hormones

43. An instrument for viewing objects that cannot be seen with the naked eye is called…..

a. Glasses

b. Micro telescope

c. Microscope

44. Cells that have a similar structure and function are joined together to form a …….

a. Tissue

b. Gland

c. Organ

45. These are glands that secrete hormones directly into the bloodstream

a. Exocrine

b. Endocrine

c. Membranes

46. This is the stage of human development from the third month of pregnancy to birth.

    a. Fetus

    b. Feces

    c. Exocrine

47. A type of fluid that contains sperm.

    a. Urinate

    b. Pigment

    c. Semen

48. Permanent brain damage will occur if the brain is without oxygen for more than…..

    a. 3 minutes

    b. 5 minutes

    c. 7 minutes

49. This is the decrease in size or wasting away of tissue

    a. Sphincters

    b. Atrophy

    c. Menarche

50. The beginning of the menstrual cycle is called………..

    a. Menarche

    b. Menopause

    c. Embryo

51. How many types of observation are there?

    a. 5

    b. 4

    c. 2

52. What is a permanent written record of a client's progress during illness and rehabilitation?

a. Care Record

b. Incident

c. Word Root

53. This means to watch carefully and attentively

a. Observe

b. Document

c. Chart

54. What are the two types of observation?

a. Aching, Burning

b. Objective, Subjective

c. Vital Signs, Subjective

55. What indicates a group of four important indicators about the body's condition?

a. Pain

b. Vital Signs

c. Discomfort

56. What is an unexpected event that occurs in the client's home or even in the agency office?

a. Pain

b. Incident

c. Frequent Questions

57. If you don't know whether an abbreviation is acceptable, what should you do?

a. Abbreviate it anyway

b. Write the complete phrase so the record is accurate

c. Do nothing at all

58. What are the three most important responsibilities of the home care aide?

a. Observing, Reporting, Recording information correctly

b. Objective, Subjective, Vital signs

   c. Client beliefs, Cultural influences, Communication

59. What are the types of pain

   a. Aching, Miserable, Nagging

   b. Exhausting, Chronic, Burning

   c. Acute, Chronic, Phantom

60. To record information correctly you must understand the special language of medicine called

   a. Word parts

   b. Suffixes

   c. Medical terminology

61. This is the word part that is the core of the term, contains basic meaning of the word

   a. Documentation

   b. Word root

   c. Phrase

62. This is the word part attached to the beginning of the word root to modify its meaning

   a. Prefix

   b. Noun

   c. Chart

63. This means that someone tells you information that you cannot observe

   a. Subjective method

   b. Objective method

   c. None of the above

64. What means feeling sore, aching, or hurting

   a. Disabled

   b. Arthritis

   c. Pain

65. Medical terminology can originate from languages, other than English.

a. True

b. False

66. This is a state of physical, mental, and social well-being

    a. Health

    b. Anxiety

    c. Illness

67. The state of being sick or a change from the state of being healthy.

    a. Mourn

    b. Anxiety

    c. Illness

68. How many types of illness are there

    a. 5

    b. 3

    c. 2

69. This type of illness last sa short time; care is given at home or in the hospital

    a. Chronic

    b. Acute

    c. Severe

70. This illness lasts a long time, maybe a life-time; care is given at home, in a rehabilitation center, or in a nursing home

    a. Chronic

    b. Mild

    c. Acute

71. A person who cannot perform the normal activities of daily living is said to have a/an

    a. Illness

    b. Anxiety attack

c. Disability

72. Disabilities are classified as the following:

    a. Physical, development, anxiety

    b. Development, emotional, physical

    c. Stress, anxiety, depression

73. What type of disability affects normal growth and development?

    a. Physical

    b. Development

    c. Depression

74. This is a refusal to admit the truth.

    a. Anger

    b. Fear

    c. Denial

75. Devices used by disabled individuals to replace a missing body part is called.....

    a. Prostheses

    b. Mourn

    c. Wheelchair

76. A feeling of intense sadness is called?

    a. Illness

    b. Depression

    c. Mourn

77. This type of disability results from illness or injury to one or more body systems.

    a. Emotional

    b. Physical

    c. Developmental

78. Equipment or other items to help clients perform activities of daily living more easily are called…………..

    a. Prostheses

    b. Health

    c. Assistive devices

79. What are the basic human needs

    a. Physical, self-esteem, psychological

    b. Self-esteem, grief, mourn

    c. Physical, mental, social

80. When you note any changes in the client's condition, you must report it to the……….

    a. Nurse

    b. Doctor

    c. Patient

81. This is an unplanned and unforeseen event or circumstance

    a. Habit

    b. Accident

    c. Emergency

82. A repeated pattern of involuntary behavior or thought is called

    a. Habit

    b. Crisis

    c. Accident

83. Another word for poisonous is called

    a. Dangerous

    b. Toxic

    c. Crisis

84. Capable of catching on fire and burning is called……….

a. Emergency

b. Crisis

c. Combustible

85. A serious situation that comes suddenly and threatens life or well-being

a. Emergency

b. Elective

c. Toxic

86. Another word for broken bone is called

a. Fracture

b. Sprain

c. Dislocation

87. What are the three things to start a fire

a. Supply of oxygen, source of heat, fire

b. Fuel, source of heat, supply of oxygen

c. None of the above

88. How many times a year are you supposed to practice fire safety in your own home

a. 5

b. 1

c. 2

89. What is the number 1 cause of home fires

a. Electrical

b. Gas leaks

c. Smoking

90. The use of ……….. in the home poses great risk of fire

a. Oxygen

b. Heater

c. None of the above

91. This is the introduction of harmful organisms

    a. Disinfect

    b. Ecologically

    c. Contamination

92. Clutter, disorder, dirt, and odors are examples of

    a. Health and safety hazards

    b. Bio hazards

    c. Disinfectant

93. If there is any questions or confusions about your duties or the timing of each job, you must

    a. Keep doing you routine job

    b. Contact your supervisor

    c. Contact the client

94. This lists your responsibilities for maintaining the client's environment

    a. Duties

    b. Job

    c. Care plan

95. What is your first priority when developing a work plan

    a. Client's bedroom

    b. Client's bathroom

    c. The care of the client

96. Big cleaning jobs are your responsibility

    a. T

    b. F

97. The tub and shower are cleaned after each use

    a. T

b. F

98. Dusting and vacuuming the bedroom or clients area is an everyday task

    a. T

    b. F

99. Cleaning toilet, commode, and bathroom sink is a weekly task

    a. T

    b. F

100.　　Do not try to do everything to do everything in one day

    a. T

    b. F

101.　　One of the easiest ways to make a home look cleaner is to eliminate clutter

    a. T

    b. F

102.　　Clutter, disorder, dirt, and odors are not health and safety hazards

    a. T

    b. F

103.　　Do not throw away anything without discussing it with your client

    a. T

    b. F

104.　　This means to remove sources of food and shelter needed for pests to grow and multiply

    a. Exclusion

    b. Sanitation

    c. Contamination

105.　　Chemical that can be applied to objects to destroy germs is called

    a. Ecologically

    b. Microorganism

c. Disinfectant

106. The process by which food is taken in and used by the body is called

   a. Nutrition

   b. Energy

   c. Malnutrition

107. Food energy is measured by a unit called

   a. Unit prices

   b. Proteins

   c. Calories

108. A lack of one or more essential nutrients in the diet is called

   a. Weight loss

   b. Anorexia

   c. Deficiency

109. This is composed of fatty acids that contain carbon, hydrogen, and oxygen

   a. Calories

   b. Fats

   c. Carbohydrates

110. These are substances that are needed to maintain our health

   a. Proteins

   b. Nutrients

   c. Carbohydrates

111. What group of vitamins do vitamins A, D, E and K belong too

   a. Fat-soluble vitamins

   b. Water- soluble vitamins

c. None of the above

112. How many essential amino acids does high- quality protein contain

   a. 5

   b. 12

   c. 9

113. What provides the body's major source of energy

   a. Carbohydrates

   b. Proteins

   c. Fatty acids

114. What type of vitamin promotes growth and prevents dry skin

   a. Vitamin D

   b. Vitamin A

   c. Vitamin E

115. Thiamin, riboflavin and folic acid are under what group of vitamin

   a. Fat-soluble vitamins

   b. Water- soluble vitamins

   c. None of the above

116. This helps to heal wounds and promotes, healthy teeth, gums, bones, and skin

   a. Vitamin B12

   b. Niacin

   c. Vitamin C

117. These are chemicals that come from water and the ground

   a. Minerals

   b. Folic acid

   c. Riboflavin

118. What percent of water is the human body composed of

a. 50%

b. 60%

c. 45%

119.   Excessive water loss from the body tissue resulting from insufficient fluid intake is called

a. Anorexia

b. Malnutrition

c. Dehydration

120.   Treatment of the clients illness may include changes in the diet which is called

a. Nutritional therapy

b. Dietitian

c. None of the above

121.   This occurs when harmful organisms enter the body and grow, causing illness or disease

a. Wound

b. Infection

c. Biohazard

122.   A group of microorganisms that usually are capable of causing or producing a disease is

called

a. Pathogenes

b. Organisms

c. Nonpathogenes

123.   This are one-celled microscopic plants that multiply very quickly

a. Fungi

b. Bacteria

c. chromosome

124. This term is used when the streptococcal organism is the cause of the disease

 a. Strep infection

 b. Staphylococcus

 c. Staph infection

125. The smallest known living disease-producing organism is called

 a. Viruses

 b. Bacteria

 c. Hepatitis C

126. These are tiny plants that live on other plants or animals and can cause diseases

 a. Streptococcus

 b. Sputum

 c. Fungi

127. These are one-celled microscopic organisms that usually live in water and cause diseases

 a. Protozoa

 b. Fungi

 c. Viruses

128. A person or animal that spreads diseases to others but does not become ill is called

 a. Aerobic

 b. Carrier

 c. Reservoir

129. ………….. is coughed up from the lungs and spit out through the mouth.

 a. Anaerobic

 b. Infection

 c. Sputum

130. Infectious diseases of the liver caused by a virus and spread through contact with blood, body fluids, and/or unprotected sex

a. AIDS

b. HIV

c. Hepatitis B/C

131. These are hollow, flexible tubes made of soft plastic or rubber that can be inserted into the body to withdraw or insert fluids

a. Intravenous infusions

b. Catheters

c. Medical asepsis

132. Another word for passed from one person or place to another is called………..

a. Transmission

b. Reservoir

c. Carrier

133. These are specialized clothing or equipment worn by an employee from protection against a biohazard

a. Anaerobic

b. Uniform

c. Personal protective equipment

134. Piercing mucous membranes or skin through needle sticks, human bites, cuts, and/or scrapes could cause………..

a. Parenteral

b. Vomitus

c. Infection

135. ……………… procedure requires entering the body.

a. Intravenous

b. Invasive

c. Pathogenic

136.   The proper use of muscles to move and lift objects and maintain correct posture is called……………

    a. Transfer

    b. Ambulate

    c. Body mechanics

137.   Loss of strength and endurance is called……….

    a. Equilibrum

    b. Fatigue

    c. Illness

138.   This means the readiness of the muscle to work

    a. Fatigue

    b. Muscle tone

    c. Tendons

139.   To move the body with or without assistance, to walk is called………….

    a. Ambulation

    b. Acute

    c. Foot drop

140.   Moving a client from one place to another is called……………

    a. Shearing

    b. Helping

    c. Transfer

141.   Wasting of muscle is called………………..

    a. Weakness

    b. Illness

    c. Muscle atrophy

142.   Shortening of muscles whereby a joint becomes permanently immovable is called

   a.   Contracture

   b.   Fatigue

   c.   Shearing

143.   A device to keep the top of the bedding from resting on client's legs and feet is called

   a.   Foot drop

   b.   Bed cradle

   c.   Ambulate

144.   Part of the bone that is near the skin's surface is called

   a.   Tendons

   b.   Bony prominence

   c.   Muscle

145.   This position is also known as the dorsal recumbent position

   a.   Supine position

   b.   Prone position

   c.   Sims position

146.   This is a sitting position

   a.   Supine position

   b.   Fowler's position

   c.   Lateral position

147.   Pressure against surface of skin and skin layers as client is being moved is called

   a.   Transfer

   b.   Muscle atrophy

   c.   Shearing

148.   This is inflammation of the lungs

   a.   Pneumonia

b. Lung disease

c. Contracture

149.   Contractures can be prevented by…

a. Range of motion exercises

b. Ambulation

c. All of the above

150.   Inability to keep the foot in a normal walking position is called

a. Foot drop

b. Footboard

c. Muscle tone

SECTION FOUR

Section four is divided into six sections.

Section four (I)

1. Every state has a uniform training requirements for home health aides

True
False

2. The HHA certification process includes at least _____ of training and as much as _____ course in a state like California

    A. 65 hours, 110 hours

    B. 25 hours, 100 hours

    C. 75 hours, 120 hours

3. The purpose and goal of home care is to provide an adequate level of care in a cost-effective manner

    True
    False

4. All of the following are ways a physician can function in the home health care setting except

    A. A physician can be an evaluator of the patient health

    B. A physician can provide assistance to patient every day activities such as bathing and eating

    C. A physician can be the one who lead the team by talking more active role in patient care

5. Who decides which of the other ancillary services like physical therapists, etc are needed by the patient?

    A. Nurse

    B. CAN

    C. Doctor

6. Who uses their clinical judgment as to whether the first dose of any drug should be given at home

    A. Physical therapist

    B. Nurse

    C. Pharmacist

7. The _____ therapist creates the home exercise program to help the patient move around more

    A. Occupational

    B. Physical

    C. Speech

8. These therapist manipulate the environment of the patient to make it easier for them to function, such as widening doors, guide rails, adjusting furniture for easier travel around the house

A. Occupational therapist

B. Speech therapist

C. Respiratory therapist

9. Allowing the patient to do more by him/herself, their self-esteem increases and there is a possible decrease in the need for constant supervision

A. True

B. False

10. This therapist use wide range of communication aids and technology such as hearing aids, they also teach sign language

A. Respiratory therapist

B. Occupational therapist

C. Speech therapist

11. The _____ provides emotional and psychological support to the home care clients.

A. Pharmacist

B. Nurse

C. Social worker

12. Which of the following fulfills the personal care role for the patient

A. Social worker

B. Home health aide

C. Nurse

13. HHAs may not help in some house hold chores such as cleaning the drapes the carpet and changing bed linen

True
False

14. All of the following include common observations and documentation to be done by the HHA except

A. Blood in urine

B. Writes prescriptions

C. Changes in mental/emotional state

15. Which of the following are the key steps in the communication process and methods of communication

    A. Creation, transmission, reception, translation and response

    B. Creation, deception, regression and translation

    C. Repetition, response, transmission and creation

16. HHAs must ask 'yes' or 'no' questions if the patient has speech problems

    True
    False

17. The most effective technique for communication is the written form of communication of the documentation

    True
    False

18. What does the acronym NAHC stand for

    A. National Associate for Home Care Hospice

    B. Nation Association for Home Care Hospice

    C. National Association for Home Care Hospice

19. All of the following are ways to communicate with a client except

    A. Maintain eye contact

    B. Not observing body language

    C. Pay attention to both verbal and nonverbal cues

20. Which of the following are ways to save time for the home health care team?

    A. Stay focused

    B. Use time management building blocks

    C. Plan and manage your schedule ahead of time

    D. All of the above

Section Four (II)

1. Home health aides help clients who have diverse needs so that they feel comfortable and obtain assistance

   True

   False

2. Is it within the scope of home health aides to change simple dressing?

   Yes

   No

3. The HHAs work under the supervision of a/an……………..

   A. LVN

   B. CNA

   C. RN

4. The client family has the right to be involved when the treatment is being planned

   True

   False

5. Home health aides should not respond to the patients queries appropriately and in time

   True

   False

6. In Maslow hierarchy of needs, the first level at the bottom is

   A. Physiological level

   B. Safety level

   C. Self-esteem level

7. The second level from the bottom of the hierarchy is

    A. Physiological

    B. Self-esteem

    C. Safety

8. _____ is the third level from the bottom of hierarchy

    A. Belonging

    B. Self-actualization

    C. Safety

9. Which of the following is the top most level in the hierarchy

    A. Self-esteem

    B. Self-actualization

    C. Safety

10. Culture, lifestyle and life experience dictates what values the client and family has

    True

    False

11. Addressing some individual by their first name or by honey or sweetie may not be insultive

    True

    False

12. _____ means thinking that one's culture is superior to another person's culture

    A. Egocentrism

B. Ethnocentrism

13. Religion can play a role in the way client and family perceives illness

True

False

14. Unlicensed home care aides are usually refered to as:

A. Caregivers

B. LVNs

C. Home Health Aides

15. Home Health Aides are individuals who have gone through a state approved training program and have passed a competency test

A. True

B. False

16. Home Health Aides can prepare simple meals in the client's home.

A. True

B. False

17. The accronymn HIPAA stands for

A. Health Intrusion Practice Accounts Act.

B. Health Insurance Practice Act

C. Health Insurance Portability and Accountability Act

18. _____ is responsible for normalizing temperature of the body, generate hormones and support the sensory organs

    A. Respiratory system

    B. Integumentary system

    C. Lymphatic system

19. Which of the following is characterized by impaired cognition and loss of memory

    A. Stroke

    B. Dementia

    C. Malaria

20. Which of the following is the 5 stages of grief by Kubler-Ross

    A. Denial, recognizing, depression, acceptance, anger

    B. Repression, anger, acceptance, denial, bargaining

    C. Denial, anger, bargaining, depression, acceptance

Section Four (III)

1. Home health aides should be proficient in skills such as bed bath, tub bathing and shower bathing.
   True

   False

2. All of the following are equipment needed for bed bath except

A. Soap and water

B. Towel

C. Iodine

3. The water to give a client bed bath should be tested with your

   A. Finger tips

   B. Elbow

   C. Feet

4. The clothes should be worn beginning with the paralyzed body parts from the top to the bottom

   True

   False

5. Improvised equipment are not helpful when required equipment's are broken or not available

   True

   False

6. Personal care delivery at home entails giving personal care according to individual needs of a client.

   True

   False

7. Which of the following is not an equipment that can be used to provide care

   A. Suitcase

   B. Diapers

   C. Lifting aids

8. _____ care is characterized by healthy eating habits, appropriate lifestyle preferences and being informed on when to ask for medical assistance

A. Assist care

B. Health care

C. Self-care

9. A _____ diet will make the body strong and prevent some illnesses caused by deficiency such as anemia

A. Balance

B. Vegetarian

C. Healthy

10. Body mechanics encourages incorrect posture when using the body and reveals physical capabilities

True

False

11. The _____ is considered a powerful source of power

A. Chest

B. Abdomen

C. Thigh

12. Pulling and pushing should be preferred to lifting

True

False

13. _____ is another principle that can enable the body perform many functions

A. Exercising

B. Pulling

C. Pushing

14. Do not ask for assistance if the client has lot of weight

True

False

15. The purpose of passive range of motion is to

A. Ensure client changes range of position after a while

B. Prolong pressure on one side

C. Facilitate gentle movement to muscles and joints for daily movement

16. The _____ is the largest organ on the body

A. Hair

B. Skin

C. Nails

17. Food rich in omega three include

A. Zinc

B. Protein

C. Vitamin A and C

D. All of the above

18. There are _____ many changes of skin break down

A. 5

B. 4

C. Nails

19. In what stage is all skin thickness lost to a depression since the dermis and epidermis layer are absent

A. Final and advanced stage

B. Third stage

C. First stage

20. A _____ is a surgical opening on a body after surgery

A. Wound

B. Cut

C. Ostomy

Section Four (IV)

1. Clients should eat a variety of food from carbohydrates, protein, minerals, fats, vitamins, minerals and sugars.

    True

    False

2. Nutrients are composed of ……………….

    A. Water, minerals

    B. Proteins, fats

    C. Carbohydrates

    D. All of the above

3. _____ is important in giving the body energy, warmth and retaining heat and energy

   A. Food

   B. Blood

   C. Water

   D. Exercise

4. Plenty of _____ and _____ should be eaten to maintain good health

   A. French Fries and Chicken nuggets

   B. Fats and sugars

   C. Fruits and vegetables

5. Taking supplement is equivalent to replacing food

   True

   False

6. It is not important to discipline self to eat food in the right amount

   True

   False

7. Good nutrition can prevent some illnesses.

   True

   False

8. Weight loss cannot be easily identified

   True

   False

9. The deficiency of nutrients hinders healing of _____ and contribute to low immune system

    A. food

    B. Wounds

    C. water

10. Aspiration pneumonia results when food gets into the lungs instead of the stomach

    True

    False

11. _____ diets refer to foods that are modified to meet the specific health and physical needs of a client

    A. Therapeutic

    B. Balanced

    C. Nutritional

12. Therapeutic diet include food low in

    A. Cholesterol

    B. Low fat

    C. Both a and b

13. Patient with diabetes mellitus have inadequate insulin and should have certain nutrients according to their specific requirements

    True

    False

14. Diabetics should have foods rich in sugars

    True

    False

15. Food poisoning can be avoided by preparing and storing food in a clean safe environment and using clean water

    True

    False

16. Food should be kept away from contamination and at recommended temperature

    True

    False

17. Enteral feeding is commonly known as _____ feeding

    A. Spoon

    B. Tube

18. Tube feeding is _____ and allows the caregivers to give nutritional supplements

    A. Safe

    B. Unsafe

19. Lack of fluid could cause constipation

    True

    False

20. The food and nutrition service in the United States help distribute excess food from farms to the needy

    True

False

Section Four (V)

1. The role of home health aide includes helping in bath, dressing, and toileting

   True

   False

2. In some cases, HHA educates the client and family when it comes to maintaining a safe clean and health environment

   True

   False

3. To maintain a safe environment, cabinets with dangerous substances and tools should be locked

   True

   False

4. Naked flames should be left unattended

   True

   False

5. A working telephone is not necessary in case of an emergency

   True

   False

6. Avoid sitting or standing too close to the patient when they cough or have flu

   True

False

7. Gloves must be worn at all times when handling soiled linen, equipment or clothes

   True

   False

8. Hands should be washed before and not after completing task

   True

   False

9. When cleaning the kitchen, start with throwing out the garbage

   True

   False

10. If there is no vacuum cleaner, sweep the carpet with a brush

    True

    False

11. When cleaning the floor what should be done first

    A. Mop

    B. Sweep

    C. Dry floor

12. When washing and drying utensils it is not important to establish if there is any utensils that need sterilization

    True

    False

13. Utensils should be sort according to types of dirt

True

False

14. Utensils should be cleaned in cold soapy water using a soft dish cloth

True

False

15. _____ Before laundering client's clothes, check for...........

A. Laundry instructions

B. Running water

C. Food in the microwave

16. Household tasks begin with a list

True

False

17. Household tasks can be sorted and arranged according to time

True

False

18. Activities can be grouped into daily, weekly and monthly tasks

True

False

19. Rooms can be cleaned once times a week

True

False

20. The dishes would take more time to clean than the fan

True

False

Section Four (VI)

1. Recent study proved that there has been a high level of growth within home care system

   True

   False

2. As of 2011 home care represented just 4 % of the total health care expenditures as compared to over 31% of total health care expenditures

   True

   False

3. Home health care is intended to grow 2.5 % in the coming decade

   True

   False

4. It is necessary to understand some of the key principles that exist within home care

   True

   false

5. Infection can be considered to be……

   A. Invasion of host organism's bodily tissues by disease-causing organisms

   B. their multiplication

C. The reaction of the host tissues to these organisms and the toxins they produce

D. All of the above

6. Some of the infections within home care encompasses broad range of issues, some are of more life threatening to health than others

   True

   False

7. Which of the following federal standards of cleanliness must hospitals comply with?

   A. Cleanliness and procedures for disposal of an array of disease causing agents

   B. Regularly schedule cleanings

   C. All of the above

8. The most common type of infection in home care is urinary tract infection

   True

   False

9. Staphylococcus aureus and enterococcus is the least type of skin infection encountered in home care

   True

   False

10. Studies have shown 6 % infection rates of the home care patients to have reported urinary tract infections and skin infections.

    True

    False

11. Health care professionals should not attempt to recognize key symptoms of infections

True

False

12. The means of infection transmission cannot be attributed to contact in one shape or form with a contaminated object or organism

True

False

13. Which of the following are modes of transmission?

    A. Contact (direct or indirect)

    B. Contaminated object or organism

    C. All of the above

14. There are many different disease carrying agents that exist within the home as to the ones found in the hospital

True

False

15. Most caregivers think that the pathogens found in the home are somehow harmless because the patient has been exposed to them their entire life.

True

False

16. Pointing out to the family that methods of harboring infection include dirty plates not washed on time and dirty linens being reused over and over is a bad idea.

True

False

17. HHAs must not wear gloves when changing diapers

True

False

18. Personal protective equipment used in the hospital setting cannot or should not be used in a home health care setting

True

False

19. The acronym PPE mean

A. Private protection equipment

B. Personal protective equipment

C. People personal protected equipment

20. Sterilization can only take place in a hospital

True

False

Section One Answers

1) A
2) D
3) A
4) D
5) C
6) D
7) B
8) B
9) B
10) C

11) A
12) B
13) C
14) D
15) D
16) B
17) D
18) B
19) A
20) B
21) C
22) D
23) A
24) C
25) D
26) B
27) A
28) D
29) C
30) B
31) C
32) A
33) A
34) A
35) D
36) C
37) D
38) C
39) C
40) D
41) A
42) C
43) D
44) C
45) D
46) C
47) B
48) A
49) D
50) D
51) D
52) B
53) C
54) A
55) B
56) C
57) D
58) True
59) A
60) B
61) D

62) B
63) A
64) A
65) A
66) B
67) D
68) B
69) A
70) D
71) D
72) A
73) D
74) B
75) B
76) A
77) C
78) C
79) D
80) A
81) A
82) D
83) D
84) B
85) D
86) C
87) A
88) A
89) B
90) D
91) D
92) C
93) A
94) D
95) D
96) B
97) C
98) D
99) A
100) A

Section Two

1. A
2. B
3. C
4. B

5. B
6. C
7. A
8. B
9. A
10. B
11. A
12. A
13. B
14. C
15. C
16. A
17. B
18. C
19. B
20. A
21. C
22. B
23. B
24. A
25. C
26. B
27. C
28. B
29. A
30. B
31. A
32. C
33. B
34. A
35. B
36. A
37. C
38. B
39. A
40. B
41. A
42. A
43. C
44. A
45. C
46. B
47. A
48. B

49. A
50. A

Section Three

1. C
2. B
3. A
4. B
5. C
6. A
7. B
8. C
9. C
10. A
11. B
12. C
13. A
14. B
15. C
16. C
17. A
18. B
19. B
20. C
21. A
22. C
23. B
24. B
25. A
26. C
27. B
28. T
29. A
30. T
31. B
32. C
33. A
34. C
35. B
36. C

37. A
38. B
39. B
40. A
41. C
42. B
43. C
44. A
45. B
46. A
47. C
48. C
49. B
50. A
51. C
52. A
53. A
54. B
55. B
56. B
57. B
58. A
59. C
60. C
61. B
62. A
63. A
64. C
65. B
66. A
67. C
68. C
69. B
70. A
71. C
72. B
73. B
74. C
75. A
76. B
77. B
78. C
79. A
80. B

81. B
82. A
83. B
84. C
85. A
86. A
87. B
88. C
89. C
90. A
91. C
92. A
93. B
94. C
95. C
96. F
97. T
98. F
99. F
100.   T
101.   T
102.   F
103.   T
104.   B
105.   C
106.   A
107.   C
108.   C
109.   B
110.   B
111.   A
112.   C
113.   A
114.   B
115.   B
116.   C
117.   A
118.   B
119.   C
120.   A
121.   B
122.   C
123.   B
124.   A

125.   A
126.   C
127.   A
128.   B
129.   B
130.   C
131.   B
132.   A
133.   C
134.   A
135.   B
136.   C
137.   B
138.   B
139.   A
140.   C
141.   C
142.   A
143.   B
144.   B
145.   A
146.   B
147.   C
148.   A
149.   C
150.   A

SECTION FOUR (I)

1. False
2. C
3. True
4. B
5. C
6. C
7. B
8. A
9. True
10. C
11. C
12. B
13. False
14. B
15. A
16. True
17. True

18. C
19. B
20. D

SECTION FOUR (II)

1. True
2. Yes
3. C
4. True
5. False
6. A
7. C
8. A
9. B
10. True
11. False
12. B
13. True
14. A
15. C
16. A
17. C
18. B
19. B
20. C

SECTION FOUR (III)

1. True
2. C
3. B
4. True
5. False
6. True
7. A
8. C
9. C
10. False
11. B
12. True
13. A
14. False

15. C
16. B
17. D
18. B
19. B
20. C

SECTION FOUR (IV)

1. True
2. D
3. A
4. C
5. False
6. False
7. True
8. False
9. B
10. True
11. A
12. C
13. True
14. False
15. True
16. True
17. B
18. A
19. True
20. True

SECTION FOUR (V)

1. True
2. True
3. True
4. False
5. False
6. True
7. True
8. False
9. False
10. True

11. B
12. False
13. True
14. False
15. A
16. True
17. True
18. True
19. False
20. True

SECTION FOUR (VI)

1. True
2. False
3. True
4. True
5. D
6. True
7. C
8. True
9. True
10. True
11. False
12. False
13. C
14. True
15. True
16. False
17. False
18. False
19. B
20. True

OTHER TITLES FROM THE SAME AUTHOR:

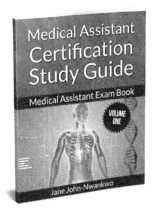

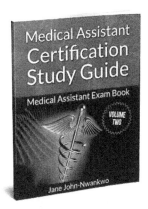

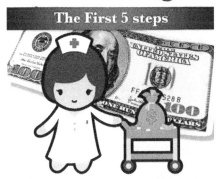

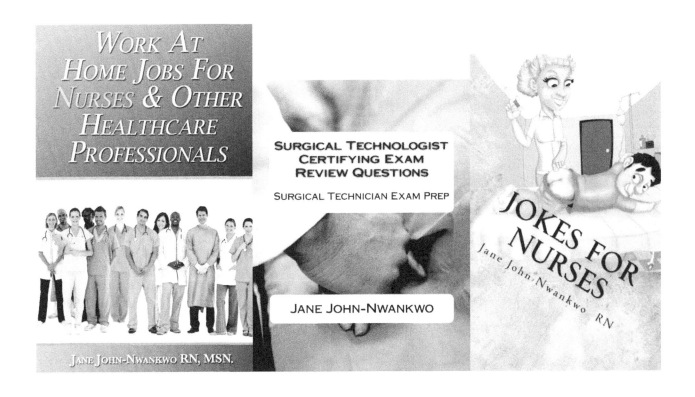

Made in the USA
Middletown, DE
23 July 2023

35503775R00053